Table of Contents

Welcome!

30 day Success plan will help you kick start your fitness goals with this rapid weight loss system, real research real goals, and practical solutions can now be yours with the Done Deal meal plan and success booklet. I've done the research and will assist in giving you the tools to be successful. I've made this very simple for beginners but made sure it was powerful enough for the advanced user So stay focused and share your results.

@ donedeal.successplan@gmail.com

General Rules

- All ingredients should be available at your local grocery store
- BCAA'S may be added after your workouts
- Recipes with Venison may be interchanged with ground beef and turkey
- Dinners may be switched or repeated except for day 5,12,19,26
- All condiments should be no lager than a tablespoon
- Please try to avoid carbonated sodas and other beverages with a high sugar content
- Meals should be eaten 3-4 hours apart
- Drink a gallon of water a day will be very beneficial to this meal plan

Disclaimer

This routine may be too extreme to do for more than 30 days at a time; Please switch to a more basic method for two or three weeks to let your body rest. This plan is considered to be a general guide to help you lose weight and may not be suitable for everyone. Please evaluate the workout regiment and meal plan with your doctor or physician before starting to make sure that you will not encounter any health problems while on the 30-day success plan Done Deal!

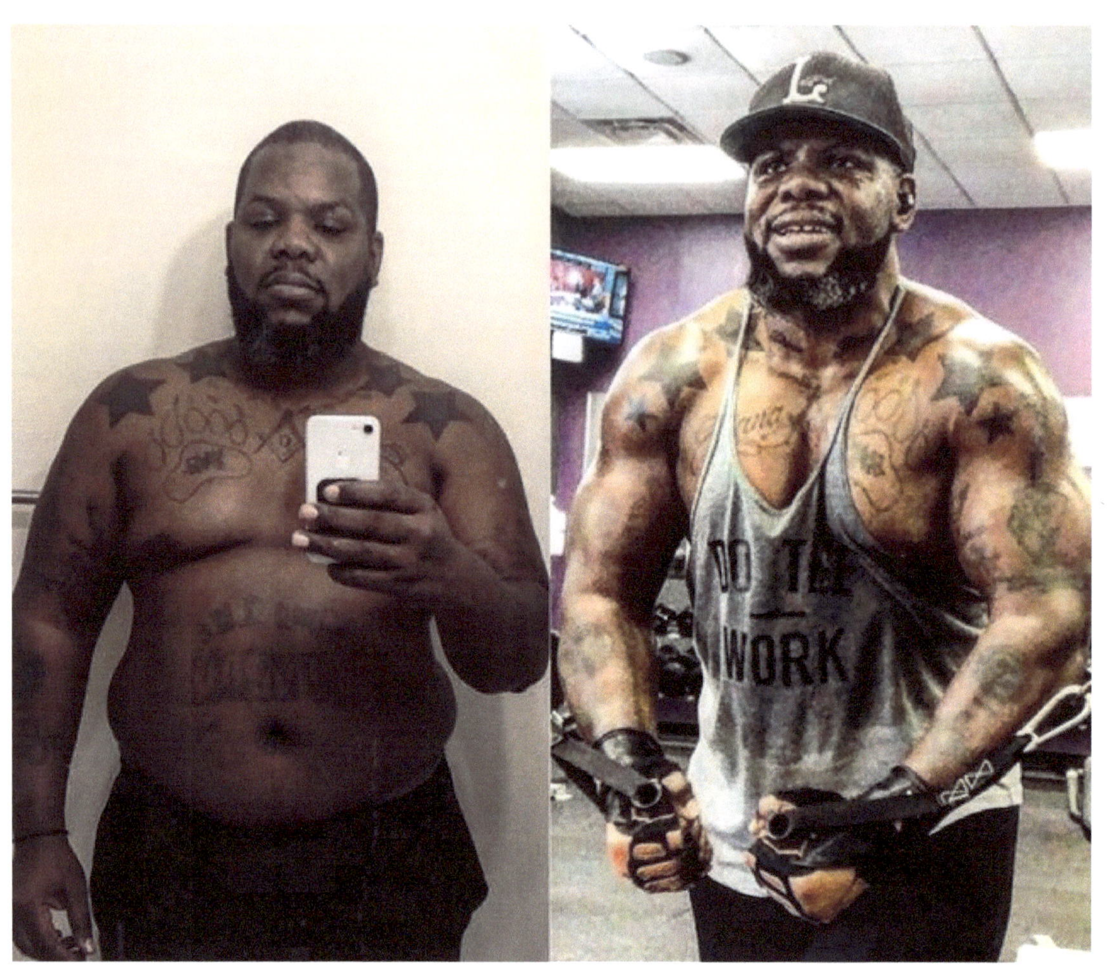
DO THE
WORK

WORKOUT A –Upper Body	
10-minute Treadmill walk	5-10 Incline
Dumbbell Bench Press (Using weight that would be difficult to achieve 16-17 reps with)	3 sets 0f 15 reps
Seated Barbell Shoulder Press (Using weight that would be difficult to achieve 16-17 reps with)	3 sets 0f 15 reps
Lat Pull Down (Using weight that would be difficult to achieve 16-17 reps with)	3 sets 0f 15 reps
Row Machine or Bent over Barbell Rows (Using weight that would be difficult to achieve 16-17 reps with)	3 sets 0f 15 reps
Rear Delt Fly Superset with Peck Deck (Using weight that would be difficult to achieve 20-22-reps with)	3 sets 0f 15 reps
Side Lateral Raise (Using weight that would be difficult to achieve 16-17 reps with)	3 sets 0f 15 reps
30-minute Treadmill Walk (Hold on if you need to but try and let your legs do the work)	Max Incline

WORKOUT B –Lower Body	
10-minute Stationary Bike	Moderate Intensity
Barbell Back Squats (Using weight that would be difficult to achieve 16-17 reps with)	2 sets 0f 15 reps
Leg Curls (Using weight that would be difficult to achieve 16-17 reps with)	4 sets 0f 15 reps
Calf Raises (Using weight that would be difficult to achieve 16-17 reps with)	3 sets 0f 15 reps
Bench Step-ups (Per leg, no additional weight)	3sets 0f 25 reps
Body Weight Squats	3 sets 0f 20 reps
30 Minute Treadmill walk (Hold on if you need to but try and let your legs do the work)	Max incline

<table>
<tr><td colspan="2" style="background-color:yellow">WORKOUT C —Core and Cardio</td></tr>
<tr><td>10-minute Treadmill walk
Incline</td><td>5-10</td></tr>
<tr><td>Core Circuit</td><td>repeat 5 times</td></tr>
<tr><td>Planks
(Core Circuit)</td><td>30seconds</td></tr>
<tr><td>Flutter Kicks
(Core Circuit)</td><td>30seconds</td></tr>
<tr><td>Weighted Cable Crunches
(Core Circuit)</td><td>10 reps</td></tr>
<tr><td>BenchJackknives
(Core Circuit)</td><td>20 reps</td></tr>
<tr><td>Jumping Jacks
(Core Circuit)</td><td>15 reps</td></tr>
<tr><td>15-minute Elliptical intervals
(Go all out for 30 seconds, slow back down to a moderate speed, and repeat Done Deal!)</td><td>Max Incline</td></tr>
</table>

All Exercises can be viewed on several web sites

https://www.bodybuilding.com/exercises/

Day 1	Breakfast	Snack	Lunch	Dinner	Late snack
	Coffee (black w/small amount of sweetener or water 1 cup of oats ½ cup of yogurt Cinnamon may be added to flavor the Oats	1 scoop of Whey Protein	6-8 Ounces of fish and a decent amount of vegetables	6-8 ounces of chicken 1 cup of rice preferably brown	Fresh fruit or ½ cup of cottage cheese

Workout-A: Upper body see workout routines in the front of the booklet

Supplement
Pre-workout
1 -2 scoops
with water

Day 2	Breakfast	Snack	Lunch	Dinner	Late snack
	Coffee (black w/small amount of sweetener or water 1 cup of oats ½ cup of yogurt Cinnamon may be added to flavor the Oats	1 scoop of Whey Protein	6-8 Ounces of fish and a decent amount of vegetables	6-8 ounces of chicken 1 cup of rice preferably brown	Fresh fruit or ½ cup of cottage cheese

Workout-B: Lower Body see workout routines in the front of the booklet

Supplement
Pre-workout
1 -2 scoops
with water

Day 3	Breakfast	Snack	Lunch	Dinner	Late snack
	Coffee (black w/small amount of sweetener or water 1 cup of oats ½ cup of yogurt Cinnamon may be added to flavor the Oats	1 scoop of Whey Protein	6-8 Ounces of fish and a decent amount of vegetables	6-8 ounces of chicken 1 cup of rice preferably brown	Fresh fruit or ½ cup of cottage cheese

Workout-C: Core and Cardio see workout routines in the front of the booklet

Supplement
Pre-workout
1 -2 scoops
with water

Day 4	Breakfast	Snack	Lunch	Dinner	Late snack
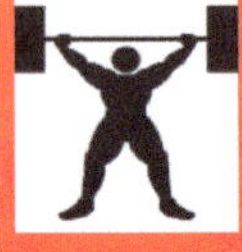	Coffee (black w/small amount of sweetener or water 1 cup of oats ½ cup of yogurt Cinnamon may be added to flavor the Oats	1 scoop of Whey Protein	6-8 Ounces of fish and a decent amount of vegetables	6-8 ounces of chicken 1 cup of rice preferably brown	Fresh fruit or ½ cup of cottage cheese
	Workout-A: Upper body see workout routines in the front of the booklet	**Supplement** Pre-workout 1 -2 scoops with water			

Day 5	Breakfast	Snack	Lunch	Dinner	Late snack
	Coffee (black w/small amount of sweetener or water 1 cup of oats ½ cup of yogurt Cinnamon may be added to flavor the Oats	1 scoop of Whey Protein	6-8 Ounces of fish and a decent amount of vegetables	Cheat Meal Medium size portions	Fresh fruit or ½ cup of cottage cheese
	Workout-B: Lower Body see workout routines in the front of the booklet	**Supplement** Pre-workout 1 -2 scoops with water			

Day 6	Breakfast	Snack	Lunch	Dinner	Late snack
	Coffee (black w/small amount of sweetener or water 1 cup of oats ½ cup of yogurt Cinnamon may be added to flavor the Oats	1 scoop of Whey Protein	6-8 Ounces of fish and a decent amount of vegetables	6-8 ounces of chicken 1 cup of rice preferably brown	Fresh fruit or ½ cup of cottage cheese
	Workout-C: Core and Cardio see workout routines in the front of the booklet	**Supplement** Pre-workout 1 -2 scoops with water			

Day 7	Breakfast	Snack	Lunch	Dinner	Late snack
	Coffee (black w/small amount of sweetener or water 1 cup of oats ½ cup of yogurt Cinnamon may be added to flavor the Oats	1 scoop of Whey Protein	6-8 Ounces of fish and a decent amount of vegetables	6-8 ounces of chicken 1 cup of rice preferably brown	Fresh fruit or ½ cup of cottage cheese
	REST, RELAX AND RECOVER	**Mentally**	**Prepare**	**For another fat-burning week**	

Day 8	Breakfast	Snack	Lunch	Dinner	Late snack
	Coffee (black w/small amount of sweetener or water 1 cup of oats ½ cup of yogurt Cinnamon may be added to flavor the Oats	1 scoop of Whey Protein	6-8 Ounces of fish and a decent amount of vegetables	6-8 ounces of Turkey 1 cup of rice preferably brown	Fresh fruit or ½ cup of cottage cheese
	Workout-A: Upper Body see workout routines in the front of the booklet	**Supplement** Pre-workout 1 -2 scoops with water			

Day 9	Breakfast	Snack	Lunch	Dinner	Late snack
	Coffee (black w/small amount of sweetener or water 1 cup of oats ½ cup of yogurt Cinnamon may be added to flavor the Oats	1 scoop of Whey Protein	6-8 Ounces of fish and a decent amount of vegetables	6-8 ounces of Turkey 1 cup of rice preferably brown	Fresh fruit or ½ cup of cottage cheese
	Workout-B: Lower Body see workout routines in the front of the booklet	**Supplement** Pre-workout 1 -2 scoops with water			

Day 10	Breakfast	Snack	Lunch	Dinner	Late snack
	Coffee (black w/small amount of sweetener or water 1 cup of oats ½ cup of yogurt Cinnamon may be added to flavor the Oats	1 scoop of Whey Protein	6-8 Ounces of fish and a decent amount of vegetables	6-8 ounces of Turkey 1 cup of rice preferably brown	Fresh fruit or ½ cup of cottage cheese
	Workout-C: Core and Cardio see workout routines in the front of the booklet	**Supplement** Pre-workout 1 -2 scoops with water			

Day 11	Breakfast	Snack	Lunch	Dinner	Late snack
	Coffee (black w/small amount of sweetener or water 1 cup of oats ½ cup of yogurt Cinnamon may be added to flavor the Oats	1 scoop of Whey Protein	6-8 Ounces of fish and a decent amount of vegetables	6-8 ounces of Turkey 1 cup of rice preferably brown	Fresh fruit or ½ cup of cottage cheese
	Workout-A: Upper Body see workout routines in the front of the booklet	**Supplement** Pre-workout 1 -2 scoops with water			

Day 12	Breakfast	Snack	Lunch	Dinner	Late snack
	Coffee (black w/small amount of sweetener or water 1 cup of oats ½ cup of yogurt Cinnamon may be added to flavor the Oats	1 scoop of Whey Protein	6-8 Ounces of fish and a decent amount of vegetables	Cheat Meal Medium size portions	Fresh fruit or ½ cup of cottage cheese
	Workout-B: Lower Body see workout routines in the front of the booklet	**Supplement** Pre-workout 1 -2 scoops with water			

Day 13	Breakfast	Snack	Lunch	Dinner	Late snack
	Coffee (black w/small amount of sweetener or water 1 cup of oats ½ cup of yogurt Cinnamon may be added to flavor the Oats	1 scoop of Whey Protein	6-8 Ounces of fish and a decent amount of vegetables	6-8 ounces of chicken 1 cup of rice preferably brown	Fresh fruit or ½ cup of cottage cheese
	Workout-C: Core and Cardio see workout routines in the front of the booklet	<u>**Supplement**</u> Pre-workout 1 -2 scoops with water			

Day 14	Breakfast	Snack	Lunch	Dinner	Late snack
	Coffee (black w/small amount of sweetener or water 1 cup of oats ½ cup of yogurt Cinnamon may be added to flavor the Oats	1 scoop of Whey Protein	6-8 Ounces of fish and a decent amount of vegetables	6-8 ounces of chicken 1 cup of rice preferably brown	Fresh fruit or ½ cup of cottage cheese
	REST, RELAX AND RECOVER	**Mentally**	**Prepare**	**For another fat-burning week**	

Day 15	Breakfast	Snack	Lunch	Dinner	Late snack
	Coffee (black w/small amount of sweetener or water 1 cup of oats ½ cup of yogurt Cinnamon may be added to flavor the Oats	1 scoop of Whey Protein	6-8 Ounces of fish and a decent amount of vegetables	6-8 ounces of chicken 1 cup of rice preferably brown	Fresh fruit or ½ cup of cottage cheese
	Workout-A: Upper Body see workout routines in the front of the booklet	<u>**Supplement**</u> Pre-workout 1 -2 scoops with water			

Day 16	Breakfast	Snack	Lunch	Dinner	Late snack
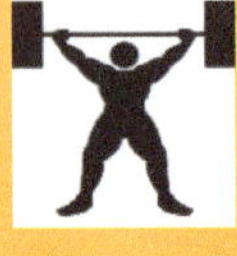	Coffee (black w/small amount of sweetener or water 1 cup of oats ½ cup of yogurt Cinnamon may be added to flavor the Oats	1 scoop of Whey Protein	6-8 Ounces of fish and a decent amount of vegetables	6-8 ounces of lean ground beef 1 cup of rice OR 1 cup Vegetables	Fresh fruit or ½ cup of cottage cheese

Workout-B: Lower Body see workout routines in the front of the booklet

<u>**Supplement**</u>
Pre-workout
1 -2 scoops
with water

Day 17	Breakfast	Snack	Lunch	Dinner	Late snack
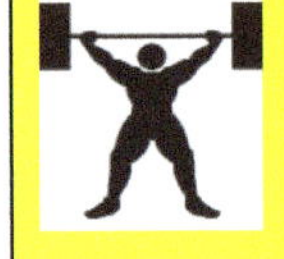	Coffee (black w/small amount of sweetener or water 1 cup of oats ½ cup of yogurt Cinnamon may be added to flavor the Oats	1 scoop of Whey Protein	6-8 Ounces of fish and a decent amount of vegetables	6-8 ounces of lean ground beef 1 cup of rice OR 1 cup Vegetables	Fresh fruit or ½ cup of cottage cheese

Workout-C: Core and Cardio see workout routines in the front of the booklet

<u>**Supplement**</u>
Pre-workout
1 -2 scoops
with water

Day 18	Breakfast	Snack	Lunch	Dinner	Late snack
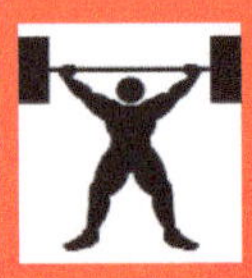	Coffee (black w/small amount of sweetener or water 1 cup of oats ½ cup of yogurt Cinnamon may be added to flavor the Oats	1 scoop of Whey Protein	6-8 Ounces of fish and a decent amount of vegetables	6-8 ounces of Steak 1 cup of rice OR 1 cup Vegetables	Fresh fruit or ½ cup of cottage cheese

Workout-A: Upper Body see workout routines in the front of the booklet

<u>**Supplement**</u>
Pre-workout
1 -2 scoops
with water

Day 19	Breakfast	Snack	Lunch	Dinner	Late snack
	Coffee (black w/small amount of sweetener or water 1 cup of oats ½ cup of yogurt Cinnamon may be added to flavor the Oats	1 scoop of Whey Protein	6-8 Ounces of fish and a decent amount of vegetables	Cheat Meal Medium size portions	Fresh fruit or ½ cup of cottage cheese
	Workout-B: Lower Body see workout routines in the front of the booklet	<u>**Supplement**</u> Pre-workout 1 -2 scoops with water			

Day 20	Breakfast	Snack	Lunch	Dinner	Late snack
	Coffee (black w/small amount of sweetener or water 1 cup of oats ½ cup of yogurt Cinnamon may be added to flavor the Oats	1 scoop of Whey Protein	6-8 Ounces of fish and a decent amount of vegetables	6-8 ounces of chicken 1 cup of rice preferably brown	Fresh fruit or ½ cup of cottage cheese
	Workout-C: Core and Cardio see workout routines in the front of the booklet	<u>**Supplement**</u> Pre-workout 1 -2 scoops with water			

Day 21	Breakfast	Snack	Lunch	Dinner	Late snack
	Coffee (black w/small amount of sweetener or water 1 cup of oats ½ cup of yogurt Cinnamon may be added to flavor the Oats	1 scoop of Whey Protein	6-8 Ounces of fish and a decent amount of vegetables	6-8 ounces of chicken 1 cup of rice preferably brown	Fresh fruit or ½ cup of cottage cheese
	REST, RELAX AND RECOVER	**Mentally**	**Prepare**	**For another fat-burning week**	

Day 22	Breakfast	Snack	Lunch	Dinner	Late snack
	Coffee (black w/small amount of sweetener or water 1 cup of oats ½ cup of yogurt Cinnamon may be added to flavor the Oats	1 scoop of Whey Protein	6-8 Ounces of fish and a decent amount of vegetables	6-8 ounces of chicken or turkey 1 cup of rice preferably brown	Fresh fruit or ½ cup of cottage cheese
	Workout-A: Upper body see workout routines in the front of the booklet	**Supplement** Pre-workout 1 -2 scoops with water			

Day 23	Breakfast	Snack	Lunch	Dinner	Late snack
	Coffee (black w/small amount of sweetener or water 1 cup of oats ½ cup of yogurt Cinnamon may be added to flavor the Oats	1 scoop of Whey Protein	6-8 Ounces of fish and a decent amount of vegetables	6-8 ounces of chicken or turkey 1 cup of rice preferably brown	Fresh fruit or ½ cup of cottage cheese
	Workout-B: Lower Body see workout routines in the front of the booklet	**Supplement** Pre-workout 1 -2 scoops with water			

Day 24	Breakfast	Snack	Lunch	Dinner	Late snack
	Coffee (black w/small amount of sweetener or water 1 cup of oats ½ cup of yogurt Cinnamon may be added to flavor the Oats	1 scoop of Whey Protein	6-8 Ounces of fish and a decent amount of vegetables	6-8 ounces of chicken or turkey 1 cup of rice preferably brown	Fresh fruit or ½ cup of cottage cheese
	Workout-C: Core and Cardio see workout routines in the front of the booklet	**Supplement** Pre-workout 1 -2 scoops with water			

Day 25	Breakfast	Snack	Lunch	Dinner	Late snack
	Coffee (black w/small amount of sweetener or water 1 cup of oats ½ cup of yogurt Cinnamon may be added to flavor the Oats	1 scoop of Whey Protein	6-8 Ounces of fish and a decent amount of vegetables	6-8 ounces of chicken or turkey 1 cup of rice preferably brown	Fresh fruit or ½ cup of cottage cheese

Workout-A: Upper body see workout routines in the front of the booklet

<u>Supplement</u>
Pre-workout
1 -2 scoops
with water

Day 26	Breakfast	Snack	Lunch	Dinner	Late snack
	Coffee (black w/small amount of sweetener or water 1 cup of oats ½ cup of yogurt Cinnamon may be added to flavor the Oats	1 scoop of Whey Protein	6-8 Ounces of fish and a decent amount of vegetables	Cheat Meal Medium size portions	Fresh fruit or ½ cup of cottage cheese

Workout-B: Lower Body see workout routines in the front of the booklet

<u>Supplement</u>
Pre-workout
1 -2 scoops
with water

Day 27	Breakfast	Snack	Lunch	Dinner	Late snack
	Coffee (black w/small amount of sweetener or water 1 cup of oats ½ cup of yogurt Cinnamon may be added to flavor the Oats	1 scoop of Whey Protein	6-8 Ounces of fish and a decent amount of vegetables	6-8 ounces of chicken or turkey 1 cup of rice preferably brown	Fresh fruit or ½ cup of cottage cheese

Workout-C: Core and Cardio see workout routines in the front of the booklet

<u>Supplement</u>
Pre-workout
1 -2 scoops
with water

Day 28	Breakfast	Snack	Lunch	Dinner	Late snack
	Coffee (black w/small amount of sweetener or water 1 cup of oats ½ cup of yogurt Cinnamon may be added to flavor the Oats	1 scoop of Whey Protein	6-8 Ounces of fish and a decent amount of vegetables	6-8 ounces of Steak 1 cup of rice OR 1 cup Vegetables	Fresh fruit or ½ cup of cottage cheese
	REST, RELAX AND RECOVER	**Mentally**	**Prepare**	**For another fat-burning week**	

Day 29	Breakfast	Snack	Lunch	Dinner	Late snack
	Coffee (black w/small amount of sweetener or water 1 cup of oats ½ cup of yogurt Cinnamon may be added to flavor the Oats	1 scoop of Whey Protein	6-8 Ounces of fish and a decent amount of vegetables	6-8 ounces of chicken or turkey 1 cup of rice preferably brown	Fresh fruit or ½ cup of cottage cheese
	Workout-A: Upper Body see workout routines in the front of the booklet	**Supplement** Pre-workout 1 -2 scoops with water			

Day 30	Breakfast	Snack	Lunch	Dinner	Late snack
	Coffee (black w/small amount of sweetener or water 1 cup of oats ½ cup of yogurt Cinnamon may be added to flavor the Oats	1 scoop of Whey Protein	6-8 Ounces of fish and a decent amount of vegetables	6-8 ounces of chicken or turkey 1 cup of rice preferably brown	Fresh fruit or ½ cup of cottage cheese
	Workout-B: Lower Body see workout routines in the front of the booklet	**Supplement** Pre-workout 1 -2 scoops with water			

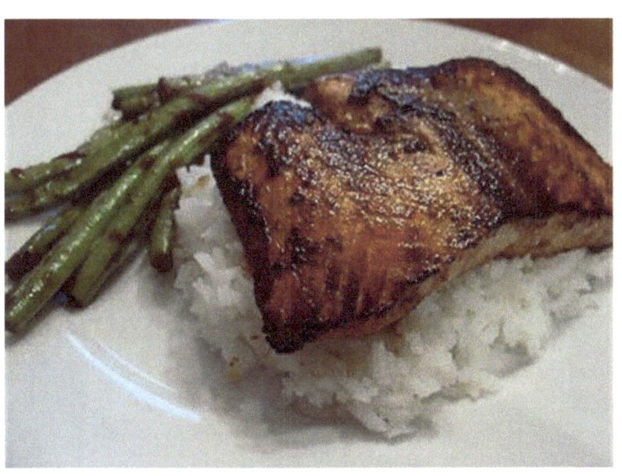

Ingredients:

2lbs salmon filets (cleaned)

¼ cup of reduced-sodium soy or coconut soy sauce

1 tablespoon of chili sauce

1 tablespoon of fresh ginger (minced)

2 cloves fresh garlic (minced)

1 lime juiced and zested

1 tablespoon of brown sugar

3 green onions diced

nstrutions:

1. Heat skillet to high heat place salmon on a cutting board.
2. In a bowl, mix soy sauce, chili sauce ginger, garlic, lime juice lime zest and brown sugar. Pour the sauce over the salmon place salmon in skillet.
3. Cook the salmon for 4-7 minutes on each side or until fully cooked. Remove and plate with side dish if there's any sauce leftover pour over salmon and top with the green onions.

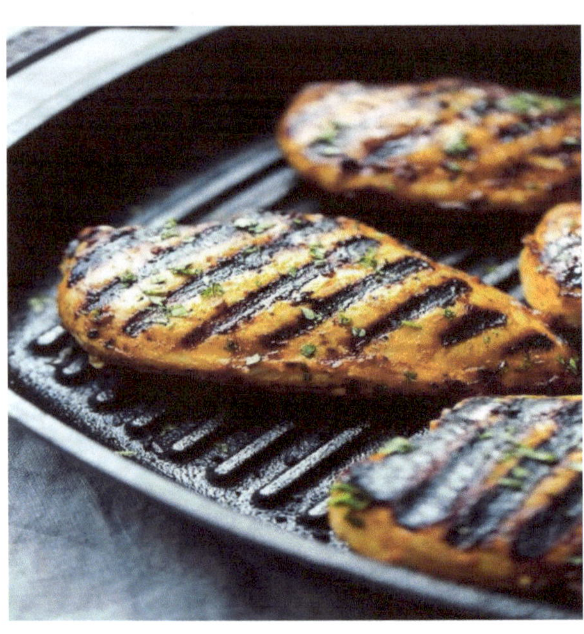

<u>Ingredients:</u>

⅓ cup soy sauce

⅓ cup brown sugar

2 tablespoons lime juice

2 tablespoons orange juice

1 tablespoon thai-style sweet chili sauce

1 teaspoon chile-garlic sauce (such as Sriracha®)

3 cloves garlic (minced)

¼ teaspoon curry powder

4 boneless chicken thighs (skinless)

<u>Instrutions:</u>

1.Place the soy sauce, brown sugar, lime juice, orange juice, sweet chili sauce, chili-garlic sauce, garlic, and curry powder in a large plastic zipper bag. Seal and knead the bag with your fingers to mix all the ingredients and dissolve the sugar. Place the chicken thighs into the marinade, squeeze out the air from the bag, zip the bag closed, and refrigerate for 4 hours or overnight.

2.Preheat an outdoor grill for medium-low heat; lightly oil the grate.

3.Remove the chicken from the bag, pour the excess marinade into a small saucepan, and bring to a full boil for about 1 minute to sterilize the marinade.

4.Grill the chicken thighs until they are no longer pink in the middle and show grill marks, about 25 minutes, basting them generously with the sterilized marinade as they grill.

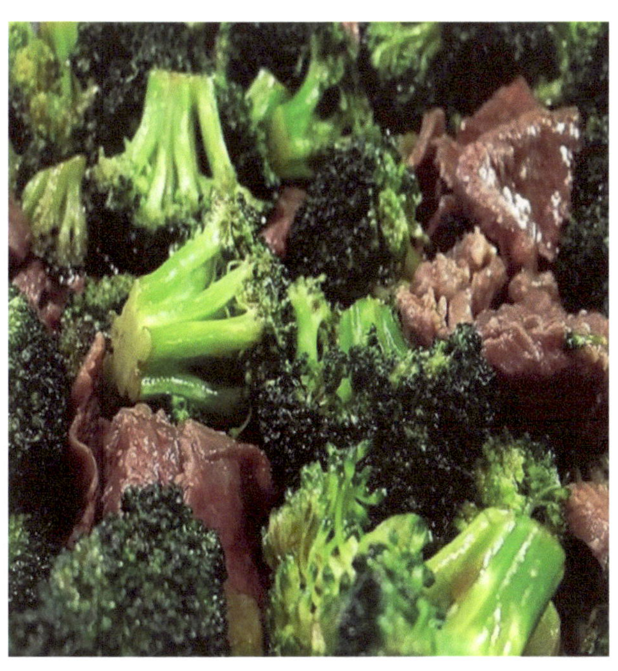

Ingredients:

⅓ cup oyster sauce

2 teaspoons Asian (toasted) sesame oil

⅓ cup sherry

1 teaspoon soy sauce

1 teaspoon white sugar

1 teaspoon cornstarch

¾ pound beef round steak, cut into 1/8-inch thick strips

3 tablespoons vegetable oil, plus more if needed

1 thin slice of fresh ginger root

1 clove garlic, peeled and smashed

1 pound broccoli, cut into florets

Instrutions:

1. Whisk together the oyster sauce, sesame oil, sherry, soy sauce, sugar, and cornstarch in a bowl and stir until the sugar has dissolved. Place the steak pieces into a shallow bowl, pour the oyster sauce mixture over the meat, stir to coat thoroughly, and marinate for at least 30 minutes in the refrigerator.

2.Heat vegetable oil in a wok or large skillet over medium-high heat, and stir in the ginger and garlic. Let them sizzle in the hot oil for about 1 minute to flavor the oil, then remove and discard. Stir in the broccoli, and toss and stir in the hot oil until bright green and almost tender, 5 to 7 minutes. Remove the broccoli from the wok and set aside.

3.Pour a little more oil into the wok, if needed, and stir and toss the beef with the marinade until the sauce forms a glaze on the meat, and the meat is

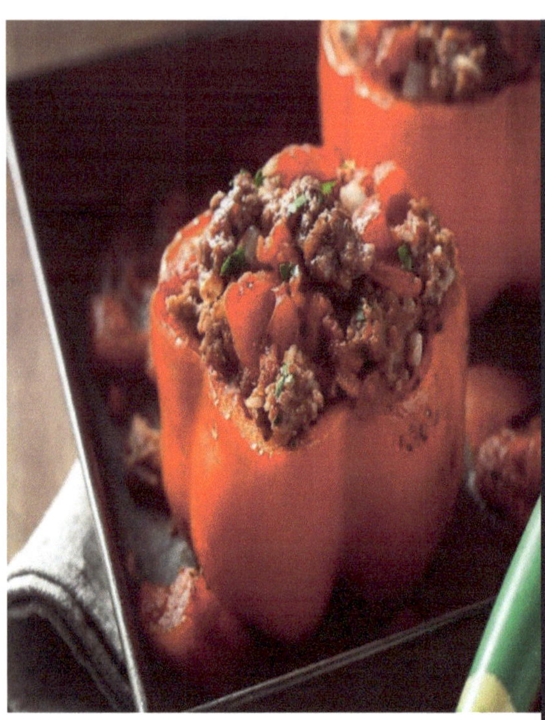

Ingredients:

1 pound Ground Beef (93% lean or leaner)

4 medium red, yellow or green bell peppers

1/2 cup minced onion

2 teaspoons minced garlic

1 can (14-1/2 ounces) diced tomatoes with green peppers and onions, drained

1/2 cup cooked white or brown rice

3 tablespoons tomato paste

2 teaspoons dried parsley leaves

1/2 teaspoon salt

1/4 teaspoon black pepper

Chopped fresh parsley leaves

Instrutions:

1. Coat a large baking dish with cooking spray; set aside. Heat oven to 475°F. Cut tops off bell peppers; set tops aside. Using a paring knife, carefully remove the membranes and seeds from bell peppers. Arrange peppers about 2 inches apart in prepared baking dish. Place tops on empty peppers. Cover baking dish tightly with aluminum foil; bake 15 minutes. Remove from oven; cool slightly.
2. Meanwhile, heat large nonstick skillet over medium heat until hot. Add ground beef, onion and garlic; cook 3 to 4 minutes, breaking beef into 1/2 inch crumbles and stirring occasionally. Stir in tomatoes, rice, tomato paste, dried parsley, salt and black pepper; cook 3 to 4 minutes until heated through, stirring occasionally.
3. Remove pepper tops. Divide beef mixture evenly among peppers; replace tops. Bake in 475°F oven 17 to 22 minutes until bell peppers are tender.

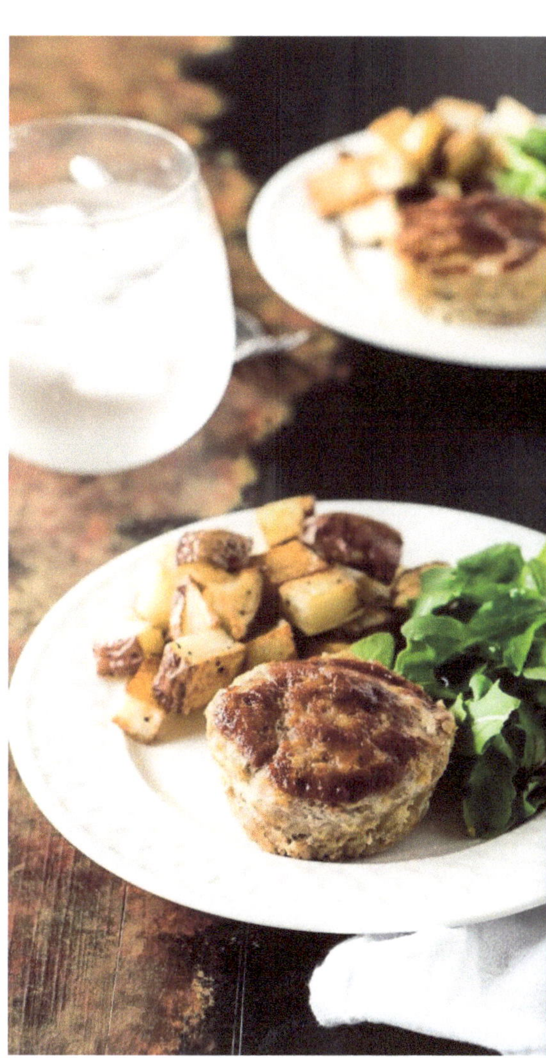

Ingredients:

1¼ lb (20 ounce) lean ground turkey (recommend using lean instead of very lean so it will be too dry)

½ teaspoon olive oil

⅓ cup diced onions

1 large egg, beaten

⅓ cup seasoned breadcrumbs (regular or gluten free)

½ teaspoon garlic powder

½ teaspoon salt

¼ teaspoon black pepper

1 teaspoon Worcestershire sauce (can sub soy sauce)

few shakes of dried oregano

3 Tablespoons ketchup, divided

3 Tablespoons BBQ sauce, divided

Instrutions:

1. Preheat oven to 350 degrees.
2. Spray a nonstick muffin tray with cooking spray or olive oil, or line it with foil or silicone liners.
3. In a small saucepan over medium heat, add olive oil and diced onions. Sauté for a 3-4 minutes then transfer to a large bowl.
4. Add ground turkey, beaten eggs, bread crumbs, garlic powder, salt, pepper, Worcestershire sauce, 1 tablespoon of ketchup and 1 tablespoon of bbq sauce. Mix together well.
5. Scoop ⅓ cup of meat mixture and fill muffin pan coated in cooking spray (will fill 8 muffin cups). Mix remaining 2 tablespoons of ketchup with 2 tablespoons of barbecue sauce. Using a spoon, divide evenly among mini meatloaves.
6. Bake for 30 minutes. Let the loaves stand in the pan for 5-10 minutes before removing. Serve with additional barbecue sauce and/or tabasco. Yield 8 mini meatloaves.

Weight Loss Log [Women]

Start Weight: ___________
Start Date: ___________
Goal: ___________

Day		Weight	Exe	Cal	Measure*	
Week 1	Su				Chest	
	M				Waist	
	Tu				Hips	
	W				Wrist	
	Th				Forearm	
	F				Date	_____
	Sa					
Week 2	Su				Chest	
	M				Waist	
	Tu				Hips	
	W				Wrist	
	Th				Forearm	
	F				Date	_____
	Sa					
Week 3	Su				Chest	
	M				Waist	
	Tu				Hips	
	W				Wrist	
	Th				Forearm	
	F				Date	_____
	Sa					
Week 4	Su				Chest	
	M				Waist	
	Tu				Hips	
	W				Wrist	
	Th				Forearm	
	F				Date	_____
	Sa					

Start Weight: ___________
Start Date: ___________
Goal: ___________

Day		Weight	Exe	Cal	Measure*	
Week 1	Su				Chest	
	M				Waist	
	Tu				Hips	
	W				Wrist	
	Th				Forearm	
	F				Date	_____
	Sa					
Week 2	Su				Chest	
	M				Waist	
	Tu				Hips	
	W				Wrist	
	Th				Forearm	
	F				Date	_____
	Sa					
Week 3	Su				Chest	
	M				Waist	
	Tu				Hips	
	W				Wrist	
	Th				Forearm	
	F				Date	_____
	Sa					
Week 4	Su				Chest	
	M				Waist	
	Tu				Hips	
	W				Wrist	
	Th				Forearm	
	F				Date	_____
	Sa					

Weight Loss Log [Men]

Start Weight:
Start Date:
Goal:

Day		Weight	Exe	Cal	Measure*	
Week 1	Su				Chest	
	M				Waist	
	Tu				Thigh	
	W				Arm	
	Th				Date	
	F					
	Sa					
Week 2	Su				Chest	
	M				Waist	
	Tu				Thigh	
	W				Arm	
	Th				Date	
	F					
	Sa					
Week 3	Su				Chest	
	M				Waist	
	Tu				Thigh	
	W				Arm	
	Th				Date	
	F					
	Sa					
Week 4	Su				Chest	
	M				Waist	
	Tu				Thigh	
	W				Arm	
	Th				Date	
	F					
	Sa					

Start Weight:
Start Date:
Goal:

Day		Weight	Exe	Cal	Measure*	
Week 1	Su				Chest	
	M				Waist	
	Tu				Thigh	
	W				Arm	
	Th				Date	
	F					
	Sa					
Week 2	Su				Chest	
	M				Waist	
	Tu				Thigh	
	W				Arm	
	Th				Date	
	F					
	Sa					
Week 3	Su				Chest	
	M				Waist	
	Tu				Thigh	
	W				Arm	
	Th				Date	
	F					
	Sa					
Week 4	Su				Chest	
	M				Waist	
	Tu				Thigh	
	W				Arm	
	Th				Date	
	F					
	Sa					